BATTLING INTERSTITIAL CYSTITIS

A Beginners Guide To Interstitial Cystitis: Diagnosis, Treatment, Coping & Living Well

ROGER ANDREW

Contents

Introduction

Chronic bladder inflammation is called interstitial cystitis (IC), or painful bladder syndrome (PBS). Pain, pressure, discomfort, or an urgent desire to urinate in the pelvis are all symptoms.

Conventional antibiotics are ineffective against interstitial cystitis since it is not due to a bacterial infection. Instead, this inflammation of the bladder wall is seen as a complex and poorly understood illness.

Interstitial cystitis is characterized by the following characteristics and symptoms:

• Chronic, varying degrees of pelvic pain are common among patients diagnosed with IC. Pain in the lower abdominal, pelvic, or bladder region is possible.

• Individuals with IC may have an increased need to urinate, sometimes even in the middle of the night (nocturia). In addition, they can have an unexpected and pressing desire to urinate.

• Constant pressure and the need to urinate even when the bladder is empty are symptoms experienced by many people with IC. A sensation of pressure or soreness in the bladder may accompany this need to urinate.

• Some persons with IC report that urinating causes them discomfort or a burning feeling.

• Patients with IC generally have a low urine output despite the persistent need to urinate.

• Interstitial cystitis (IC) flares are periods of increased symptom severity. Periods of remission, during which symptoms improve, may be followed by flares, during which symptoms worsen, in some people.

• Discomfort or pain during sexual activity is one way in which IC can negatively impact a person's quality of life.

Interstitial cystitis is difficult to diagnose due to the lack of knowledge about its root cause. Inflammation of the bladder, disruption of the bladder's protective lining, nerve dysfunction, and an overactive immune system are all thought to have a role.

When making a diagnosis, it's important to rule out potential causes of the symptoms being experienced.

Lifestyle adjustments, dietary modifications, physical therapy, drugs to reduce discomfort and inflammation, and, in rare situations, bladder instillations or surgeries are all potential components of an individualized treatment plan for interstitial cystitis.

Because of the chronic nature of IC treatment, a team effort between urologists, pain management specialists, and other medical professionals may be necessary.

CHAPTER ONE
Clinical Presentation And Diagnosis

Interstitial cystitis (IC) symptoms may manifest differently in each individual and may also change over time. Common signs and diagnostic criteria for IC are as follows:

IC Symptoms That You Might Experience:

• Discomfort in the Pelvis or Bladder Area Chronic discomfort in the lower abdomen, pelvis, or bladder area is a classic sign of IC. This discomfort may be minor, moderate, or severe, and it may be consistent or sporadic.

• The need to urinate more frequently is a common symptom of IC. This may involve urinating at any time of the day or night (known medically as nocturia).

• An urgent need to urinate occurs suddenly and intensely, even though the bladder is not full.

• Feelings of pressure or discomfort in the bladder or lower abdominal region may be present.

• Some people with IC report that urinating causes them discomfort or a burning feeling.

• Even though you may have to go to the bathroom frequently, you may only be able to pass a small volume of urine each time.

• Discomfort or pain during sexual activity (dyspareunia) is a common symptom of IC.

• Symptoms of IC can go through periods of remission when they get better and flares where they get worse.

Criteria for the Diagnosis of Interstitial Cystitis:

Because there is currently no reliable diagnostic test for IC, making a diagnosis might be difficult. Instead, the following criteria are used in conjunction with clinical evaluation to arrive at a diagnosis:

• Elimination of Other Conditions: Urinary tract infections, bladder cancer, endometriosis, and syphilis are all potential causes of comparable symptoms that must usually be ruled out before a diagnosis of IC can be made.

• For IC to be classified as a chronic condition, symptoms must last for at least six weeks.

• The inside of the bladder can be examined with a procedure called a cystoscopy. In this technique, the doctor examines the bladder for inflammation (glomerulations or Hunner's ulcers) using a thin, flexible tube equipped with a camera.

• When further evaluating tissue abnormalities, a cystoscopy may include a biopsy of the bladder lining.

• The patient should mention urinary frequency, urgency, and any pain or discomfort in the bladder.

• It is important for the doctor to rule out any alternative possibilities before treating the patient, as was discussed earlier.

It's crucial to remember that there is no one-and-only diagnostic sign or test for IC. Clinical suspicion, symptom presentation, and rule-out of alternative diagnoses all contribute to the final determination.

Because of the wide range of symptoms and causes of IC, it is important for the patient to work closely with their healthcare team, which may include a urologist, a pain management specialist, and a physical therapist, among others.

Effects On Happiness And Well-Being

The chronic and frequently debilitating symptoms of interstitial cystitis (IC) can have a major effect on a person's ability to enjoy life. Some people may feel the affects more strongly than others, and the intensity of symptoms might vary from person to person. The quality of life can be impacted by IC in the following ways:

• IC is characterized by persistent pelvic pain and discomfort. The severity and persistence of this discomfort can significantly diminish quality of life and make day-to-day tasks difficult.

• In addition to causing sleep disruption, having to get up multiple times throughout the night to urinate can leave you feeling drained, irritable, and less productive during the day.

• Needing to go to the bathroom immediately can be very upsetting and make it difficult to leave the house or participate in social activities.

• Intimate relationships and sexual happiness can be strained by sexual dysfunction, which includes painful sexual intercourse (dyspareunia).

• Stress, depression, and worry are all common side effects of dealing with a chronic disease like IC. Symptom flare-ups and their potential effects on everyday living might be unpredictable, which can exacerbate mental health concerns.

• Isolation: Because of the unpredictable nature of symptom flares and the need for frequent bathroom stops, some people with IC may withdraw socially. This may lead to less interactions with others and even estrangement from loved ones.

• Productivity at Work: Symptoms of IC may cause decreased output in the office. Reduced productivity and the potential for promotion may result from the requirement for regular breaks to alleviate pain and discomfort.

• Individuals with IC may experience financial hardship due to the high expense of medical care, including continuing treatment, doctor visits, and medication.

• Many persons with IC report improvement in their symptoms after making dietary modifications including eliminating particular foods and drinks. This can make it hard for them to eat out with friends and family.

• Difficulties in Treatment: IC management frequently necessitates a team effort involving medication, physical therapy, and behavioral adjustments. It can be a trial-and-error process to find appropriate medications, and some people may not respond well to the currently available therapy.

Individuals with IC should collaborate closely with their healthcare professionals to create a treatment plan that is tailored to their unique set of symptoms and needs. Counseling and support groups can also assist people with IC deal with the emotional and psychological challenges of daily life.

Although IC can have a serious effect on quality of life, many people are able to alleviate their symptoms and live better lives with the help of medicinal interventions, behavioral modifications, and social support. Despite the difficulties caused by IC, people can still live meaningful lives with the support of early diagnosis and proper care.

CHAPTER TWO

Learning About Your Urinary System

Production, storage, and excretion of urine are all handled by the urinary system, sometimes called the renal system. Waste products are removed from the circulation, hydration and electrolyte balance are preserved, and blood pressure is controlled. Key urinary system components and their respective roles are outlined below.

• The kidneys, which are bean-shaped structures on either side of the spine immediately below the rib cage, are the key organs of the urinary system. The kidneys' primary job is to generate urine by filtering blood of waste products and surplus substances like water and salts. There are millions of nephrons, or filtering units, in each kidney.

• Kidney function is maintained by specialized cells called nephrons. The kidneys are made up of renal tubules and renal corpuscles. The renal tubule processes the filtrate formed by the renal corpuscle to create urine. Nephrons are essential for regulating the concentrations of fluids and electrolytes in the blood.

• Connecting each kidney to the bladder are muscular tubes called ureters. Peristaltic contractions aid in the downward movement of urine as it travels from the kidneys to the bladder.

• The bladder is an organ in the pelvis that is both hollow and muscular. Urine is collected and held there until it can be flushed out of the body. Because of its elastic nature, the bladder can store a wide range of urine volumes.

• The tube that leads from the bladder to the outside world is called the urethra. Urine leaves the body through this opening. The urethra of males is longer than that of females so that it can transport semen during the ejaculatory process.

The Urinary System and What It Does:

• The kidneys perform a blood filtration process, clearing the blood of toxins, extra electrolytes, and water. A highly concentrated liquid, called filtrate, is the end result of this procedure.

• Renal tubules are responsible for reabsorbing glucose, electrolytes, and water from the filtrate back into the bloodstream, among other vital compounds.

• The kidneys produce chemicals like hydrogen ions and medicines into the urine to regulate the body's pH and flush out waste.

• The kidneys control the concentration of urine according to how well the body is hydrated. Urine becomes more concentrated when the body is trying to conserve water. Diluted urine is the effect of drinking too much water.

• The kidneys' renin-angiotensin-aldosterone system is responsible for a large portion of blood pressure regulation through its effects on blood volume and vasoconstriction.

• The active form of vitamin D, which is required for calcium absorption and bone health, is metabolized in part by the kidneys.

• Urine, the byproduct of the urinary system's operations, is expelled from the body via the urethra after traveling from the bladder. This aids in the processing of metabolic waste and preserving the steady state.

The urinary system is essential for the body's health and homeostasis because it controls the balance of fluids, eliminates waste, and aids in many metabolic processes. Urinary system dysfunction is associated with numerous medical complications and may necessitate therapeutic intervention to rectify.

Interstitial Cystitis: What Causes It And What Triggers It

Interstitial cystitis (IC) is a disorder that affects the urinary tract, but its precise causes are unknown. Several hypotheses have been proposed as to what may cause or set off IC, but none have been verified. It's vital to keep in mind that IC is a highly individual illness, with different people reacting differently to different stimuli. Some possible causes and precipitating factors of IC are as follows:

• One popular explanation proposes that IC is linked to a problem with the bladder's lining (epithelium). Inflammation of the bladder lining may result if irritating compounds in urine are able to pass through this hole.

• Researchers have hypothesized that the inflammatory and painful symptoms of IC could be the result of an autoimmune reaction in which the body's immune system wrongly targets the bladder's tissues.

• There may be a connection between IC and abnormalities in the nerves that regulate bladder function. A heightened sensitivity to bladder fullness pain and other aberrant feelings may result from these disorders.

• Although IC is not an illness, a previous bladder infection or injury may bring on the condition in certain people. Inflammation and symptoms may be brought on by damage to the bladder lining caused by infections or trauma.

• Genetics: IC tends to run in families, suggesting a possible hereditary susceptibility.

• Some people with IC experience a worsening of their symptoms during times of hormonal change, such as before and during menstruation.

• Some people find that their IC symptoms are made worse by the meals and drinks they consume. Foods high in capsaicin, caffeine, alcohol, citrus fruits, and artificial sweeteners can all set off an allergic reaction. Keeping a food diary can be a useful tool for figuring out what foods cause reactions in an individual.

• Although stress is not a direct cause of IC, it is known to exacerbate the symptoms of the condition in some people.

• Some people with IC find that intense physical activity or certain activities that place pressure on the pelvic area bring on symptoms.

• Some people with IC may experience a worsening of their symptoms after being exposed to chemicals or irritants in the environment or in their own personal care products.

Keep in mind that IC is a diagnosis of exclusion; in other words, it cannot be diagnosed until all other possible explanations for the symptoms have been exhausted. Clinical assessment, symptom history, cystoscopy, and the ruling out of other possible causes are frequently used in making a diagnosis.

Dietary and lifestyle changes, symptom-relieving drugs, physical therapy, and, in rare circumstances, surgical procedures are all part of the multidisciplinary approach used to treat inflammatory bowel disease (IC).

Quality of life can be improved for those with IC through tailored treatment that targets their specific symptoms and triggers and, in some cases, requires continuing maintenance.

CHAPTER THREE
Alternative Treatments

Interstitial cystitis (IC) treatment typically targets symptom reduction and quality of life enhancement for those who suffer from the ailment. What works for one person with IC may not work for another, therefore it's crucial to recognize that IC treatment is generally personalized. Some potential approaches to treating IC are:

1. Alterations to One's Way of Life and Diet:

• Dietary Modifications: Many people who suffer from IC find relief when they cut out caffeine, alcohol, spicy foods, citrus fruits, and artificial sweeteners from their diet.

• Water helps dilute pee, making it less irritating to the bladder, therefore it's important to drink enough of water throughout the day.

• Some people find that increasing the amount of time that passes between urinations and decreasing urgency is helped by engaging in bladder training.

2. Chiropractic care:

• Physical treatment for the pelvic floor may be prescribed to assist reduce stress and enhance the performance of the pelvic floor muscles, both of which can exacerbate IC symptoms.

3. Medications:

• Oral Medications: Depending on the patient's symptoms, doctors may recommend oral medications such antihistamines, tricyclic antidepressants, pain relievers, or pentosan polysulfate sodium (Elmiron) to help repair the bladder lining.

• Bladder instillations: a method of administering medication by placing the medication directly into the bladder via catheter. Instillation drugs such as dimethyl sulfoxide (DMSO) and heparin are often utilized.

• Some people receive relief from lidocaine or a rescue instillation, which are both topical drugs administered directly to the bladder walls.

4. Stimulating a Nerve:

• Surgery called sacral neuromodulation includes implanting a device (neurostimulator) to control bladder function by stimulating the sacral nerves. In some circumstances, it may be useful for symptom management.

5. Botulinum toxin (Botox) injections into the bladder wall have been shown to relax the bladder, hence decreasing urinary urgency and frequency in some patients.

6. Surgery: When all other therapies have failed, surgery may be considered. Bladder augmentation, urinary diversion, and cystectomy are all surgical procedures that can be used to treat overactive bladder. These are usually reserved for emergency situations because of the high risk of consequences.

7. Some people try out alternative treatments, including acupuncture or herbal pills, to enhance their conventional medical care. Consult your doctor before attempting any of these alternatives.

8. Psychological Care: The persistent pain and distress associated with IC can have a major effect on a person's emotional well-being. Emotional elements of life with IC can be better managed with the use of psychosocial support, such as therapy or support groups.

It can take time and multiple attempts to determine the optimal treatment plan for a person with irritable bowel syndrome (IC). In order to improve the patient's quality of life, a healthcare expert, typically a urologist or urogynecologist, will work closely with the patient to create a customized treatment plan.

People with IC must keep an open line of contact with their medical staff in order to monitor their condition and make any required adjustments to their treatment plan.

Controlling The Effects Of Intermittent Confinement

Modifying one's lifestyle, eating habits, receiving medical care, and employing self-care techniques are all potential components of symptom management for interstitial cystitis (IC). To improve one's quality of life and lessen their suffering are the primary goals. The following are some methods for alleviating the signs of IC:

1. Changes in the Diet:

• To learn which meals and drinks are aggravating your condition, keep a food diary. Caffeine, alcohol, citrus fruit, spicy foods, artificial sweeteners, and acidic foods are common allergens.

• Consider switching to a low- or no-irritant diet if you suffer from irritable bowel syndrome (IC). The "bladder diet," which emphasizes eating foods that are gentler on the bladder, could be one such strategy.

• Stay Hydrated: Urine might be less irritating to the bladder if it is diluted by drinking enough of water throughout the day.

2. Medications:

• Consult your doctor about any drugs that could help reduce your symptoms. • Medications used to heal the bladder lining include pentosan polysulfate sodium (Elmiron), antihistamines, tricyclic antidepressants, and pain medications.

• It's possible that your doctor will suggest a topical treatment or bladder instillations to help.

3. Controlling Your Bladder:

• Keep your bladder from getting too full, which can increase discomfort, by going to the bathroom frequently.

• Deep breathing and other relaxation techniques can help ease muscle tension and bladder irritation, and can be used as part of a bladder relaxation routine.

4. Chiropractic care:

• If you think that tight muscles or dysfunction in your pelvic floor could be causing or exacerbating your symptoms, you may want to look into pelvic floor physical therapy.

5. Reducing Stress:

• Try some stress-reduction methods out, like yoga, meditation, or deep breathing. The symptoms of IC might be made worse by stress.

6. Personal Care and Hygiene:

• Soaps, bubble baths, and scented hygiene products might irritate the genital area, therefore it's best to avoid using them.

• Loose-fitting clothes restricts blood flow, so wear cotton underwear instead.

7. Heat Treatment:

• If you're experiencing pain or discomfort in your lower abdominal or pelvic area, try using a heating pad or warm compress there.

8. Be mindful of how much liquids you drink, as both dehydration and overhydration can make your symptoms worse. Finding a happy medium is crucial.

9. Drug Administration:

• Take any drugs, such as Elmiron or any recommended for your condition, exactly as directed by your doctor.

10. Mutual Aid Societies:

• If you're struggling emotionally due to having a chronic ailment, you may want to join an IC support group or see a therapist.

11. Please Seek the Advice of Your Physician:

• Schedule consistent follow-up visits with your doctor so he or she may assess your progress and make any necessary adjustments to your therapy.

12. Complementary therapy such as acupuncture, biofeedback, and dietary supplements provide help for some people. Before attempting any of these, talk to your doctor.

It's important to keep in mind that it may take some time to find the best combination of treatments for treating IC symptoms. It's critical to keep lines of communication open with your doctor and take an active role in your care.

Symptoms of IC can be better managed and your quality of life enhanced with the help of a multidisciplinary healthcare team that includes a urologist, a pain management specialist, a physical therapist, and a counselor.

CHAPPTER FOUR
Managing Interstitial Cystitis In Daily Life

Interstitial cystitis (IC) is a painful bladder illness that has no known cure. However, many people with IC may successfully manage their symptoms and keep their quality of life high with the help of appropriate measures and support. Some suggestions for coping with IC are as follows.

• Get an education; it will give you freedom of choice. Get as much information as you can on IC, including as its symptoms, causes, and treatments. If you have a firm grasp of your health situation, you can make educated decisions about your treatment.

• Create a safety net by leaning on your friends and loved ones when you need some extra assistance. If you feel like you need to talk to someone who understands what you're going through, look into IC support groups, either in person or online.

• Keep an Open Line of contact with Your Doctor Make sure you keep an open line of contact with your doctor, who should be a urologist or urogynecologist. Talk to your doctor about your symptoms, worries, and potential treatments. If you feel you need a second opinion, don't be afraid to get one.

• If you want to control your IC, it's important to stick to the treatment plan prescribed by your doctor. Alterations to one's diet, medication, physical therapy, and other treatments may be necessary. When dealing with symptoms, consistency is essential.

• Maintain a notebook to record your symptoms, their onset, and any associated events or triggers. You and your doctor can use this information to zero in on the most beneficial changes you can make to your diet and routine.

• Reduce your stress levels; it may make your IC symptoms worse. Meditation, yoga, deep breathing exercises, and mindfulness practices are just some of the stress-reduction methods you can incorporate into your daily life.

• Modifying Your DietBe on the lookout for foods and drinks that may aggravate your condition, and try to steer clear of them. Try several foods that are safe for people with IC and see what works best for you.

• Avoid dehydration and over hydration by maintaining a steady fluid intake. Be aware of your urination schedule and any underlying causes when you increase your water intake.

• Personal Hygiene Pick mild, unscented soaps and shampoos to avoid skin irritation. Keep your apparel loose and airy with cotton underwear.

10.Take care of your bladder by frequently emptying it and never holding in urine for long periods of time.

• Maintain a regular schedule of low-impact exercise as recommended by your doctor. Physical activity has been shown to enhance health and decrease anxiety.

• When your symptoms flare up, try using a heating pad or warm compress to your lower stomach or pelvic area.

• If you need to use the restroom frequently while traveling or out with friends, make sure you schedule frequent breaks and pack any essential medications or supplies.

• Therapy or counseling might help you deal with the emotional struggles of living with a chronic condition.

• Do what you can to help yourself; take an active role in your medical care. Do not be afraid to express your concerns or lack of progress with treatment to your healthcare provider.

• Understand that IC management is a continual process with potential highs and lows, and adjust your expectations accordingly. Instead of trying to find a cure, you should work on enhancing your quality of life and coping with your symptoms.

Many people with IC manage to live happy and productive lives despite the difficulties that come with dealing with the condition.

You can learn to live well with IC by coordinating your treatment with your medical professionals, making any required changes to your lifestyle, and reaching out for emotional and social support from those around you.

Conclusion

Interstitial cystitis (IC) is a chronic bladder ailment that can have serious consequences for a person's daily life. Although the precise origins of IC are unknown, it is thought to be due to a number of factors working together, such as abnormalities in the bladder's lining, immunological reactions, neurological issues, and others. Lifestyle adjustments, dietary changes, medications, physical therapy, and self-care measures all have a role in IC management.

While having IC can be difficult, many people are able to successfully manage their symptoms via treatment, social support, and knowledge. Finding the optimal combination of measures to increase comfort, lessen pain, and enhance health requires close collaboration with healthcare practitioners, open lines of communication, and patience.

Remember that you are not alone if you or someone you know has IC. Having access to emotional and practical help through resources like support groups, counseling, and a solid support network is essential. With hard work and support, people with IC can manage the difficulties of their disease and live fulfilling lives.

THE END